LOW SODIUM COOKBOOK FOR CONGESTIVE HEART FAILURE

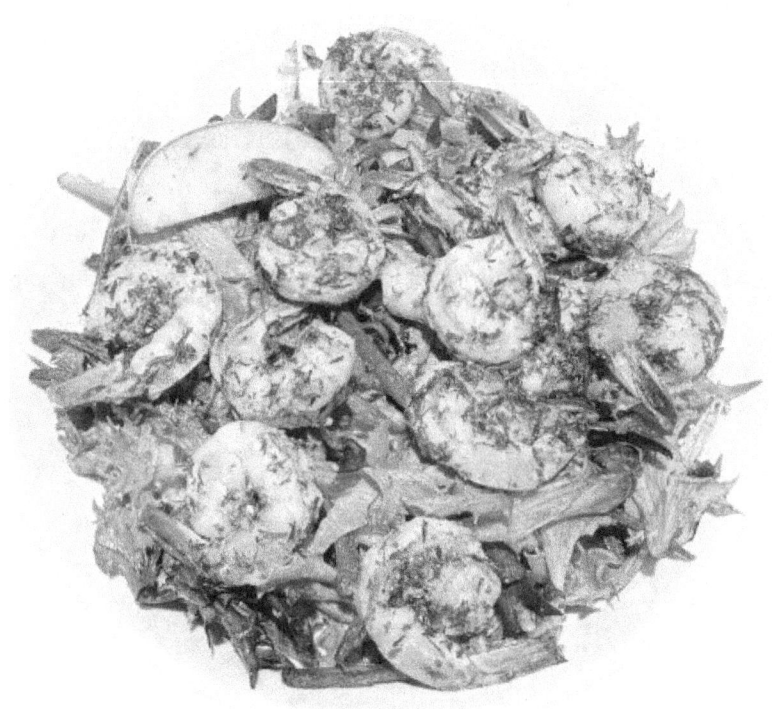

LORENE PEACHEY

DISCLAIMER

The content within this book reflects my thoughts, experiences, and beliefs. It is meant for informational and entertainment purposes. While I have taken great care to provide accurate information, I cannot guarantee the absolute correctness or applicability of the content to every individual or situation. Please consult with relevant professionals for advice specific to your needs.

TABLE OF CONTENTS

INTRODUCTION

In the heartland of America, where the sun paints the vast landscapes in warm hues, and the breeze whispers tales of comfort, I stumbled upon a culinary journey that not only saved lives but also added a dash of flavour to them. My name is Lorene Peachey, a nutritionist on a mission to unravel the secrets of a low-sodium cookbook that transformed not just the way we eat, but the way we live. This is the story of how my cookbook, with a twist as unique as an Appalachian sunrise, became the beacon of hope for those battling congestive heart failure.

A quaint little town named Maplewood, tucked away in the hills of West Virginia, where hearty laughter echoed through the valleys. In the heart of this town lived a remarkable woman named Loretta Honeycutt. Loretta, with her bright eyes and a spirit as resilient as the mountains that surrounded her, had been struggling with congestive heart failure for years. She had tried every cookbook on the market, hoping to find a solution that would bring her comfort without sacrificing the joy of savouring a good meal.

"I've been on this rollercoaster of diets, my dear. I've tried bland, tasteless meals that made my taste buds weep, and I've experimented with exotic ingredients that left me more confused than satisfied," Loretta confided in me during one of our nutrition sessions.

Her eyes gleamed with a flicker of hope as she asked, "Lorene, is there no salvation for my taste buds? Can't I enjoy a hearty meal without worrying about the consequences?"

Little did she know that the answer was about to arrive at her doorstep in the form of a cookbook with a name as charming as a southern drawl— "LOW SODIUM COOKBOOK FOR CONGESTIVE HEART FAILURE."

As Loretta delved into the pages of this culinary treasure trove, she discovered a world where low sodium wasn't synonymous with lacklustre taste. It was a revelation that transformed her kitchen into a haven of health and flavour. The recipes weren't just a collection of ingredients; they were a symphony of tastes that danced on her palate.

One evening, Loretta prepared the " Baked Salmon with Dill Sauce," a dish so exquisite that it could turn an ordinary dinner into a celebration of life. The aroma of herbs and spices filled her kitchen, and as she took the first bite, a smile crept across her face—a smile that radiated joy and triumph over her culinary battles.

As Loretta embraced the low-sodium lifestyle, she noticed a remarkable shift in her health. The constant struggle for breath eased, and her energy levels surged. With each passing day, she felt the grip of congestive heart failure loosening its hold on her life. The transformation was not just physical; it was a renaissance of the spirit.

Now, my dear reader, let me pose a question that lingers like the morning mist over the rolling hills: How often have you found yourself scouring through cookbooks, hoping to stumble upon a culinary oasis that not only supports your health but also tantalizes your taste buds?

Consider this cookbook not just a collection of recipes but a compass guiding you through a flavourful journey towards a healthier heart. The benefits of adopting a low-sodium diet extend beyond the confines of a medical chart. It's a choice that resonates with the very essence of life—a choice to Savor the richness of every moment without compromise.

Imagine waking up each morning with a newfound Vigor, ready to embrace the day with enthusiasm. Envision yourself indulging in meals that not only nurture your body but also invigorate your soul. The Flavors of the Heart cookbook is more than just a collection of recipes; it's a testament to the power of choice—a choice to live a life that pulsates with vitality.

Now, let's address the elephant in the room—the consequences of high sodium consumption. Close your eyes for a moment and picture a river, flowing effortlessly through the landscape, nourishing the earth, and sustaining life. Now, imagine that river turning into a raging torrent, overwhelming everything in its path. That, my friend, is the impact of high sodium on the human body.

High sodium levels act as the turbulent force that disrupts the delicate balance within. The heart, the conductor of this symphony of life, finds itself struggling against the rising tide. Congestive heart failure, like an uninvited storm, wreaks havoc on the cardiovascular system, leaving in its wake a trail of exhaustion and breathlessness.

The consequences of high sodium consumption are not confined to physical discomfort alone. They ripple through the emotional and psychological realms, casting a shadow over the simplest pleasures of life. Imagine being unable to Savor the warmth of a homemade soup or relish the delicate Flavors of a carefully crafted salad. The emotional toll of such limitations is immeasurable.

So, why choose the Flavors of the Heart cookbook? What sets it apart in this vast sea of culinary guides?

For starters, it's a guide penned with the care and expertise of a seasoned nutritionist, woven with the tales of those who have triumphed over dietary challenges. But beyond that, it's an invitation to rediscover the joy of eating. Each recipe is a chapter in the story of your health—a story that unfolds with every flavourful bite.

The advantage of having this cookbook in your hands goes beyond the realm of mere recipes. It's a roadmap to a healthier, more vibrant life—a life where the kitchen becomes a sanctuary of well-being, and every meal is a celebration of good health.

As we embark on this culinary adventure together, my dear reader, let me leave you with a final thought. Imagine a life where every meal is not just a necessity but a pleasure—an experience that nourishes both body and soul. The Flavors of the Heart cookbook is more than a collection of low-sodium recipes; it's a testament to the transformative power of choosing a path that embraces health without compromising on the joys of indulgence.

So, with a heart full of hope and a kitchen brimming with possibilities, let's embark on this journey together—a journey that promises not just a low-sodium lifestyle but a symphony of Flavors that will resonate through the corridors of your heart for years to come.

Contact the Author

Thank you for reading my book! I would love to hear from you, whether you have feedback, questions, or just want to share your thoughts. Your feedback means a lot to me and helps me improve as a writer.

Please don't hesitate to reach out to me through

lorenepeachey@gmail.com

I look forward to connecting with my readers and appreciate your support in this literary journey. Your thoughts and comments are valuable to me.

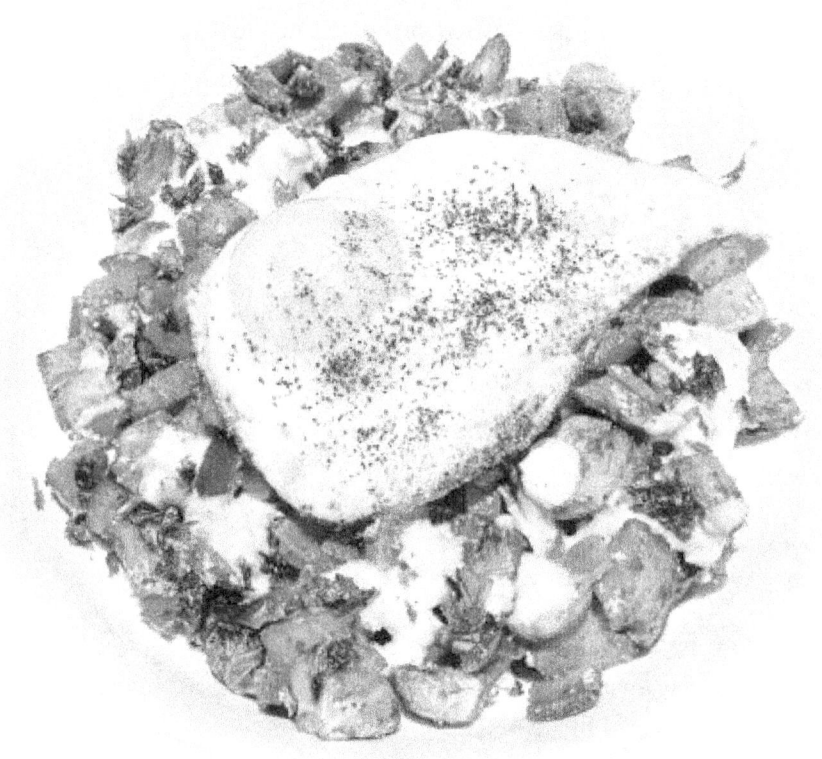

CHAPTER 1

UNDERSTANDING CONGESTIVE HEART FAILURE

Congestive Heart Failure (CHF) is a chronic condition in which the heart is unable to pump blood effectively, leading to a buildup of fluid in the lungs and other parts of the body. Managing CHF involves various lifestyle changes, and one crucial aspect is maintaining a low-sodium diet. This dietary modification plays a pivotal role in alleviating symptoms and improving the overall well-being of individuals with CHF.

Importance of a Low-Sodium Diet:

Sodium, a component of salt, is known to contribute to fluid retention in the body. For individuals with CHF, excess fluid can exacerbate heart failure symptoms, including shortness of breath, swelling, and fatigue. A low-sodium diet helps regulate fluid balance and reduces the strain on the heart, making it an essential component of managing CHF.

Reducing sodium intake is vital for controlling blood pressure, another critical factor in heart health. Elevated blood pressure can further stress the heart and worsen the progression of CHF. By adhering to a low-sodium diet, individuals can help manage their blood pressure and improve their overall cardiovascular health.

How This Cookbook Can Help:

Adopting a low-sodium diet may seem challenging, but with the right resources, it becomes more manageable. This cookbook is designed specifically for individuals with CHF, providing a diverse array of delicious and heart-healthy recipes. Here's how it can be instrumental in supporting those with CHF:

Nutrient-Optimized Recipes:

The cookbook offers recipes that are not only low in sodium but also rich in essential nutrients. It ensures that individuals with CHF receive the necessary vitamins and minerals for overall well-being while adhering to dietary restrictions.

Flavorful Alternatives:

Many people associate a low-sodium diet with bland food. However, this cookbook proves that heart-healthy meals can be both nutritious and flavorful. It introduces creative alternatives and seasonings that add taste without compromising on health.

Educational Insights:

In addition to recipes, the cookbook provides educational insights on the importance of a low-sodium diet for managing CHF. It explains how certain ingredients affect heart health and empowers individuals to make informed choices about their nutrition.

Meal Planning and Tips:

Practical tips and meal plans are included to assist individuals in seamlessly integrating a low-sodium diet into their daily lives. This resource aims to simplify the process of meal preparation, making it accessible for individuals and their caregivers.

CHAPTER 2

KEY PRINCIPLES OF LOW-SODIUM

COOKING

Reading and Understanding Food Labels:

Serving Size: Pay attention to the serving size on the label. All the information provided is based on this specified portion.

Sodium Content: Look for the sodium content per serving. Choose foods with lower sodium levels, especially if you are aiming to reduce your overall sodium intake.

Percentage Daily Value (% DV): Aim for foods with lower percentages of the Daily Value for sodium. Foods with 5% DV or less are considered low in sodium.

Ingredients List: Be wary of high-sodium additives like monosodium glutamate (MSG), sodium nitrate, and sodium benzoate. Ingredients are listed in descending order by weight, so if a high-sodium ingredient is near the top, the product likely contains more of it.

Choosing Low-Sodium Ingredients:

Fresh Produce: Focus on fresh fruits and vegetables. They are naturally low in sodium and provide essential nutrients.

Lean Proteins: Opt for lean meats, poultry, and fish. Fresh or frozen varieties without added sodium are better choices.

Whole Grains: Choose whole grains like brown rice, quinoa, and whole wheat over refined grains. They are naturally lower in sodium.

Low-Sodium or No-Salt-Added Options: Select low-sodium or no-salt-added versions of canned vegetables, beans, and broths. Rinse canned foods to reduce sodium content further.

Herbs and Spices: Use herbs, spices, and other flavorings to enhance the taste of your dishes without relying on salt.

Cooking Techniques for Flavor Without Salt:

Herbs and Spices: Experiment with herbs such as basil, thyme, oregano, and spices like cumin, paprika, and turmeric to add depth and flavor to your dishes.

Citrus Juices: Use lemon, lime, or orange juice to add a burst of freshness and acidity to your meals.

Vinegars: Balsamic vinegar, apple cider vinegar, and rice vinegar can provide tanginess without added sodium.

Garlic and Onions: These aromatic vegetables can elevate the taste of your dishes without the need for excessive salt.

Grilling and Roasting: Cooking methods like grilling and roasting intensify natural flavors, reducing the reliance on added salt.

CHAPTER 3

BREAKFAST RECIPES

Oatmeal with Berries and Almonds

Cooking Time: 10 minutes

Serving: 1

Ingredients:

- ❖ 1/2 cup old-fashioned oats
- ❖ 1 cup unsweetened almond milk
- ❖ 1/2 cup mixed berries (strawberries, blueberries, raspberries)
- ❖ 1 tablespoon chopped almonds.

Instructions:

1. Cook oats in almond milk according to package instructions.
2. Top with mixed berries and chopped almonds.

Nutritional Information:

250 calories, 40g carbs, 8g protein, 7g fat, 6g fiber.

Start your day with heart-healthy oats, packed with fiber, antioxidants from berries, and good fats from almonds.

Greek Yogurt Parfait

Cooking Time: 5 minutes

Serving: 1

Ingredients:

- ❖ 1/2 cup non-fat Greek yogurt
- ❖ 1/4 cup granola (low sodium)
- ❖ 1/2 cup fresh mango chunks
- ❖ 1 tablespoon honey

Instructions:

1. Layer yogurt, granola, and mango in a glass.
2. Drizzle with honey.

Nutritional Information:

280 calories, 45g carbs, 15g protein, 4g fat, 5g fiber.

Enjoy a protein-packed parfait with the sweetness of mango and a touch of honey for a satisfying and heart-healthy breakfast.

Avocado Toast with Poached Egg

Cooking Time: 15 minutes

Serving: 1

Ingredients:

- ❖ 1 slice whole-grain bread
- ❖ 1/2 ripe avocado
- ❖ 1 poached egg
- ❖ Salt and pepper to taste

Instructions:

1. Toast the bread and spread mashed avocado on top.
2. Place a poached egg on the avocado.

Nutritional Information:

320 calories, 25g carbs, 14g protein, 20g fat, 8g fiber.

Fuel your morning with the goodness of whole grains, healthy fats from avocado, and protein from a perfectly poached egg.

Chia Seed Pudding

Preparation Time: 5 minutes (+overnight soaking)

Serving: 1

Ingredients:

- ❖ 2 tablespoons chia seeds
- ❖ 1 cup almond milk
- ❖ 1/2 teaspoon vanilla extract
- ❖ 1/2 cup sliced strawberries.

Instructions:

1. Mix chia seeds, almond milk, and vanilla extract; refrigerate overnight.
2. Top with sliced strawberries before serving.

Nutritional Information:

200 calories, 20g carbs, 5g protein, 10g fat, 8g fiber.

Start your day with a nutrient-packed chia seed pudding, a rich source of omega-3 fatty acids and fiber.

Vegetable Egg White Omelets

Cooking Time: 10 minutes

Serving: 1

Ingredients:

- ❖ 3 egg whites
- ❖ 1/4 cup diced bell peppers.
- ❖ 1/4 cup diced tomatoes.
- ❖ 1/4 cup chopped spinach.
- ❖ 1 teaspoon olive oil

Instructions:

1. Whisk egg whites and pour into a heated, oiled pan.
2. Add vegetables, cook until set, and fold.

Nutritional Information:

150 calories, 10g carbs, 20g protein, 5g fat, 3g fiber.

Fuel your body with a protein-packed, low-calorie omelet featuring colorful veggies for added nutrients.

Banana Nut Smoothie

Preparation Time: 5 minutes

Serving: 1

Ingredients:

- ❖ 1 medium banana
- ❖ 1/2 cup unsweetened almond milk
- ❖ 2 tablespoons chopped walnuts.
- ❖ 1/2 teaspoon cinnamon

Instructions:

1. Blend banana, almond milk, walnuts, and cinnamon until smooth.

Nutritional Information:

220 calories, 30g carbs, 5g protein, 10g fat, 5g fiber.

Sip on a delicious and potassium-rich smoothie to support heart health and provide lasting energy.

Quinoa Breakfast Bowl

Cooking Time: 15 minutes

Serving: 1

Ingredients:

- ❖ 1/2 cup cooked quinoa
- ❖ 1/4 cup sliced almonds.
- ❖ 1/2 cup fresh berries (your choice)
- ❖ 1 tablespoon honey

Instructions:

1. Mix cooked quinoa with almonds.
2. Top with fresh berries and drizzle with honey.

Nutritional Information:

280 calories, 40g carbs, 8g protein, 8g fat, 6g fiber.

Elevate your morning with a quinoa bowl, providing a hearty dose of protein, fiber, and antioxidants.

Smoked Salmon and Avocado Wrap

Preparation Time: 10 minutes

Serving: 1

Ingredients:

- ❖ 1 whole-grain wrap
- ❖ 2 ounces smoked salmon.
- ❖ 1/2 avocado, sliced.
- ❖ 1 tablespoon cream cheese (low-fat)

Instructions:

1. Spread cream cheese on the wrap.
2. Layer with smoked salmon and avocado; roll up.

Nutritional Information:

300 calories, 25g carbs, 20g protein, 15g fat, 8g fiber.

Indulge in omega-3 fatty acids from smoked salmon and the creamy goodness of avocado in this delightful wrap.

Sweet Potato and Kale Hash

Cooking Time: 20 minutes

Serving: 1

Ingredients:

- ❖ 1 small, sweet potato, grated
- ❖ 1 cup chopped kale
- ❖ 1 teaspoon olive oil
- ❖ 1 poached egg

Instructions:

1. Sauté sweet potato and kale in olive oil until tender.
2. Top with a poached egg.

Nutritional Information:

280 calories, 35g carbs, 10g protein, 10g fat, 7g fiber.

Energize your morning with this nutrient-rich hash, featuring the goodness of sweet potatoes and leafy greens.

Cottage Cheese and Fruit Bowl

Preparation Time: 5 minutes

Serving: 1

Ingredients:

- ❖ 1/2 cup low-fat cottage cheese
- ❖ 1/2 cup diced pineapple.
- ❖ 1/2 cup sliced kiwi.
- ❖ 1 tablespoon chopped mint (optional)

Instructions:

1. Combine cottage cheese, pineapple, and kiwi.
2. Garnish with chopped mint if desired.

Nutritional Information:

220 calories, 30g carbs, 15g protein, 5g fat, 3g fiber.

Satisfy your taste buds with a refreshing and protein-packed cottage cheese bowl, loaded with tropical fruits.

CHAPTER 4

LUNCH AND DINNER ENTREES

Grilled Lemon Herb Chicken

Cooking Time: 20 minutes

Serving: 4

Ingredients:

- ❖ 4 boneless, skinless chicken breasts
- ❖ 2 tablespoons olive oil
- ❖ 1 lemon (juiced)
- ❖ 1 teaspoon dried oregano

Instructions:

1. Marinate chicken in olive oil, lemon juice, and oregano.
2. Grill until fully cooked.

Nutritional Information:

280 calories, 2g carbs, 35g protein, 14g fat, 1g fiber.

Enjoy a light and flavorful grilled chicken, rich in lean protein and heart-healthy olive oil.

Baked Salmon with Dill Sauce

Cooking Time: 15 minutes

Serving: 2

Ingredients:

- ❖ 2 salmon fillets
- ❖ 1 tablespoon olive oil
- ❖ 2 tablespoons fresh dill (chopped)
- ❖ 1 lemon (sliced)

Instructions:

1. Rub salmon with olive oil, top with dill and lemon slices.
2. Bake until salmon flakes easily.

Nutritional Information:

320 calories, 2g carbs, 30g protein, 20g fat, 0g fiber.

Indulge in omega-3 fatty acids with this easy-to-make baked salmon, complemented by a zesty dill sauce.

Quinoa and Vegetable Stir-Fry

Cooking Time: 15 minutes

Serving: 3

Ingredients:

- 1 cup quinoa (cooked)
- 1 cup broccoli florets
- 1 bell pepper (sliced)
- 1 carrot (julienned)
- 2 tablespoons low-sodium soy sauce

Instructions:

1. Stir-fry vegetables, add cooked quinoa, and soy sauce.
2. Cook until vegetables are tender.

Nutritional Information:

280 calories, 45g carbs, 10g protein, 8g fat, 7g fiber.

Fuel your body with a nutrient-packed quinoa stir-fry, providing a balance of protein, fiber, and essential vitamins.

Turkey and Vegetable Skewers

Cooking Time: 25 minutes

Serving: 4

Ingredients:

- ❖ 1-pound lean turkey breast, cut into cubes
- ❖ 1 zucchini, sliced.
- ❖ 1 red onion, sliced.
- ❖ 1 tablespoon olive oil

Instructions:

1. Thread turkey, zucchini, and onion onto skewers.
2. Grill until turkey is cooked through.

Nutritional Information:

240 calories, 6g carbs, 30g protein, 10g fat, 2g fiber.

Savor the goodness of lean turkey and vegetables on skewers, a delightful and low-sodium option for lunch or dinner.

Mushroom and Spinach Stuffed Chicken Breast

Cooking Time: 30 minutes

Serving: 2

Ingredients:

- ❖ 2 boneless, skinless chicken breasts
- ❖ 1 cup mushrooms (sliced)
- ❖ 1 cup fresh spinach
- ❖ 1 tablespoon olive oil

Instructions:

1. Sauté mushrooms and spinach in olive oil.
2. Stuff mixture into chicken breasts and bake until chicken is cooked.

Nutritional Information:

290 calories, 4g carbs, 35g protein, 15g fat, 3g fiber.

Elevate your dinner with this nutrient-dense stuffed chicken, a flavorful combination of lean protein and veggies.

Vegetarian Lentil Soup

Cooking Time: 40 minutes

Serving: 6

Ingredients:

- ❖ 1 cup dry lentils
- ❖ 1 onion (diced)
- ❖ 2 carrots (sliced)
- ❖ 2 celery stalks (chopped)
- ❖ 4 cups low-sodium vegetable broth

Instructions:

1. Cook lentils and vegetables in vegetable broth until tender.
2. Season to taste and serve.

Nutritional Information:

220 calories, 40g carbs, 15g protein, 1g fat, 10g fiber.

Warm your soul with a hearty lentil soup, low in sodium and high in fiber and plant-based protein.

Shrimp and Vegetable Brown Rice Stir-Fry

Cooking Time: 20 minutes

Serving: 4

Ingredients:

- ❖ 1 pound shrimp (peeled and deveined)
- ❖ 2 cups mixed vegetables (broccoli, bell peppers, snap peas)
- ❖ 2 cups cooked brown rice.
- ❖ 2 tablespoons low-sodium soy sauce

Instructions:

1. Stir-fry shrimp and vegetables, add cooked rice and soy sauce.
2. Cook until heated through.

Nutritional Information:

300 calories, 45g carbs, 20g protein, 6g fat, 7g fiber.

Satisfy your taste buds with this colorful shrimp stir-fry, a low-sodium alternative to takeout.

Chickpea and Spinach Curry

Cooking Time: 25 minutes

Serving: 4

Ingredients:

- ❖ 2 cans chickpeas (drained)
- ❖ 1 onion (chopped)
- ❖ 2 cups fresh spinach
- ❖ 1 can low sodium diced tomatoes.

Instructions:

1. Sauté onions, add chickpeas, spinach, and diced tomatoes.
2. Simmer until flavors meld.

Nutritional Information:

260 calories, 45g carbs, 15g protein, 4g fat, 10g fiber.

Delight in the flavors of a hearty chickpea and spinach curry, a plant-based dish rich in protein and fiber.

Baked Cod with Lemon and Herbs

Cooking Time: 15 minutes

Serving: 2

Ingredients:

- ❖ 2 cod fillets
- ❖ 1 tablespoon olive oil
- ❖ 1 teaspoon dried thyme
- ❖ 1 lemon (sliced)

Instructions:

1. Coat cod with olive oil, sprinkle with thyme, and top with lemon slices.
2. Bake until fish is opaque and flakes easily.

Nutritional Information:

230 calories, 2g carbs, 30g protein, 12g fat, 0g fiber.

Savor the simplicity of baked cod with the brightness of lemon and the aromatic touch of herbs.

Eggplant and Chickpea Stew

Cooking Time: 35 minutes

Serving: 4

Ingredients:

- ❖ 1 large eggplant (cubed)
- ❖ 1 can chickpeas (drained)
- ❖ 1 bell pepper (diced)
- ❖ 2 cups low-sodium vegetable broth

Instructions:

1. Combine eggplant, chickpeas, bell pepper, and vegetable broth.
2. Simmer until vegetables are tender.

Nutritional Information:

250 calories, 40g carbs, 12g protein, 5g fat, 8g fiber.

Indulge in the heartiness of an eggplant and chickpea stew, a comforting and low-sodium option for a wholesome meal.

Spinach and Feta Stuffed Turkey Burgers

Cooking Time: 25 minutes

Serving: 4

Ingredients:

- ❖ 1-pound lean ground turkey
- ❖ 2 cups fresh spinach (chopped)
- ❖ 1/2 cup crumbled feta cheese.
- ❖ 1 teaspoon garlic powder

Instructions:

1. Mix turkey, spinach, feta, and garlic powder.
2. Form into patties and grill until fully cooked.

Nutritional Information:

280 calories, 4g carbs, 30g protein, 15g fat, 2g fiber.

Elevate your burger game with these lean turkey patties stuffed with nutrient-rich spinach and feta.

Cauliflower Fried Rice with Tofu

Cooking Time: 20 minutes

Serving: 3

Ingredients:

- ❖ 1 head cauliflower (riced)
- ❖ 1 cup extra-firm tofu (cubed)
- ❖ 1 cup mixed vegetables (peas, carrots, corn)
- ❖ 2 tablespoons low-sodium soy sauce

Instructions:

1. Sauté tofu and vegetables, add cauliflower rice and soy sauce.
2. Cook until heated through.

Nutritional Information:

220 calories, 20g carbs, 15g protein, 10g fat, 6g fiber.

Enjoy a flavorful twist on classic fried rice with this cauliflower and tofu alternative, rich in plant-based goodness.

Mango Glazed Chicken Breast

Cooking Time: 30 minutes

Serving: 2

Ingredients:

- ❖ 2 boneless, skinless chicken breasts
- ❖ 1 mango (pureed)
- ❖ 1 tablespoon honey
- ❖ 1 teaspoon ginger (grated)

Instructions:

1. Mix mango puree, honey, and ginger.
2. Brush onto chicken and bake until done.

Nutritional Information:

290 calories, 25g carbs, 35g protein, 5g fat, 2g fiber.

Add a tropical flair to your meal with mango-glazed chicken, a sweet and savory delight.

Vegetable and Lentil Stuffed Bell Peppers

Cooking Time: 40 minutes

Serving: 4

Ingredients:

- ❖ 4 bell peppers (halved)
- ❖ 1 cup cooked lentils
- ❖ 1 zucchini (diced)
- ❖ 1 cup cherry tomatoes (halved)

Instructions:

1. Mix lentils, zucchini, and tomatoes.
2. Stuff into bell peppers and bake until peppers are tender.

Nutritional Information:

250 calories, 40g carbs, 15g protein, 3g fat, 10g fiber.

Indulge in a colorful and nutrient-packed meal with these stuffed bell peppers featuring lentils and fresh vegetables.

Lemon Garlic Shrimp Linguine

Cooking Time: 20 minutes

Serving: 2

Ingredients:

- ❖ 8 ounces whole-grain linguine
- ❖ 1 pound shrimp (peeled and deveined)
- ❖ 2 tablespoons olive oil
- ❖ 3 cloves garlic (minced)

Instructions:

1. Cook linguine, sauté shrimp and garlic in olive oil.
2. Toss with cooked linguine.

Nutritional Information:

320 calories, 40g carbs, 25g protein, 10g fat, 5g fiber.

Savor the flavors of a light and zesty shrimp linguine, a delightful and heart-healthy pasta option.

Stuffed Portobello Mushrooms with Quinoa

Cooking Time: 30 minutes

Serving: 3

Ingredients:

- ❖ 3 large portobello mushrooms
- ❖ 1 cup cooked quinoa
- ❖ 1 cup baby spinach (chopped)
- ❖ 1/4 cup grated Parmesan cheese.

Instructions:

1. Remove mushroom stems, mix quinoa, spinach, and cheese.
2. Stuff mushrooms and bake until tender.

Nutritional Information:

270 calories, 30g carbs, 15g protein, 12g fat, 6g fiber.

Enjoy a hearty and satisfying meal with these quinoa-stuffed portobello mushrooms, a flavorful vegetarian option.

Turkey and Vegetable Chili

Cooking Time: 40 minutes

Serving: 6

Ingredients:

- ❖ 1 pound ground turkey
- ❖ 1 onion (diced)
- ❖ 2 bell peppers (chopped)
- ❖ 1 can low-sodium black beans (drained)

Instructions:

1. Brown turkey and onions; add peppers and beans.
2. Simmer until flavors meld.

Nutritional Information:

280 calories, 25g carbs, 25g protein, 10g fat, 8g fiber.

Warm up with a comforting bowl of turkey and vegetable chili, a hearty and low-sodium option for chilly days.

Sesame Ginger Tofu Stir-Fry

Cooking Time: 25 minutes

Serving: 3

Ingredients:

- ❖ 1 block extra-firm tofu (cubed)
- ❖ 2 cups broccoli florets
- ❖ 1 red bell pepper (sliced)
- ❖ 2 tablespoons low-sodium soy sauce

Instructions:

1. Sauté tofu, broccoli, and bell pepper; add soy sauce.
2. Stir-fry until vegetables are tender.

Nutritional Information:

260 calories, 20g carbs, 20g protein, 12g fat, 5g fiber.

Experience the bold flavors of sesame and ginger in this tofu stir-fry, a delicious and nutritious alternative.

Cilantro Lime Grilled Shrimp Skewers

Cooking Time: 15 minutes

Serving: 4

Ingredients:

- ❖ 1-pound large shrimp (peeled and deveined)
- ❖ 1/4 cup fresh cilantro (chopped)
- ❖ 2 limes (juiced)
- ❖ 1 tablespoon olive oil

Instructions:

1. Marinate shrimp in cilantro, lime juice, and olive oil.
2. Skewer and grill until shrimp are opaque.

Nutritional Information:

230 calories, 5g carbs, 25g protein, 12g fat, 1g fiber.

Transport your taste buds with these zesty cilantro lime grilled shrimp skewers, a light and flavorful dish.

Mediterranean Chickpea Salad

Preparation Time: 15 minutes

Serving: 4

Ingredients:

- ❖ 2 cans chickpeas (drained)
- ❖ 1 cucumber (diced)
- ❖ 1 cup cherry tomatoes (halved)
- ❖ 1/4 cup feta cheese (crumbled)

Instructions:

1. Combine chickpeas, cucumber, tomatoes, and feta.
2. Toss with olive oil and lemon juice.

Nutritional Information:

240 calories, 35g carbs, 10g protein, 8g fat, 8g fiber.

Enjoy the vibrant flavors of the Mediterranean with this refreshing chickpea salad, a nutrient-packed and low-sodium option.

CHAPTER 5

SIDES AND SNACKS

Cucumber and Tomato Salsa

Preparation Time: 10 minutes

Serving: 4

Ingredients:

- ❖ 2 cucumbers (diced)
- ❖ 1 cup cherry tomatoes (halved)
- ❖ 1/4 red onion (finely chopped)
- ❖ 1 tablespoon fresh cilantro (chopped)

Instructions:

1. Combine cucumbers, tomatoes, onion, and cilantro in a bowl.
2. Mix well and refrigerate before serving.

Nutritional Information:

40 calories, 10g carbs, 1g protein, 0g fat, 2g fiber.

Refresh your palate with this light and vibrant cucumber and tomato salsa, a low-sodium snack bursting with flavors.

Baked Sweet Potato Fries

Cooking Time: 25 minutes

Serving: 4

Ingredients:

- ❖ 2 large, sweet potatoes (cut into fries)
- ❖ 1 tablespoon olive oil
- ❖ 1 teaspoon smoked paprika.

Instructions:

1. Toss sweet potatoes with olive oil and paprika.
2. Bake until golden and crispy.

Nutritional Information:

120 calories, 25g carbs, 2g protein, 2g fat, 4g fiber.

Indulge in guilt-free snacking with these baked sweet potato fries, offering a satisfying crunch with a hint of smokiness.

Greek Yogurt and Berry Parfait

Preparation Time: 5 minutes

Serving: 1

Ingredients:

- ❖ 1/2 cup non-fat Greek yogurt
- ❖ 1/4 cup low-sugar granola
- ❖ 1/2 cup mixed berries (strawberries, blueberries)

Instructions:

1. Layer yogurt, granola, and berries in a glass.
2. Repeat and enjoy.

Nutritional Information:

180 calories, 30g carbs, 15g protein, 2g fat, 5g fiber.

Satisfy your sweet tooth with this nutritious Greek yogurt and berry parfait, a delightful blend of textures and flavors.

Edamame and Sea Salt

Cooking Time: 5 minutes

Serving: 2

Ingredients:

- ❖ 2 cups frozen edamame (steamed)
- ❖ Sea salt to taste

Instructions:

1. Steam edamame according to package instructions.
2. Sprinkle with sea salt and toss.

Nutritional Information:

150 calories, 12g carbs, 14g protein, 7g fat, 8g fiber.

Fuel up with protein-packed edamame sprinkled with sea salt, a simple and nutritious snack to keep you energized.

Caprese Skewers

Preparation Time: 15 minutes

Serving: 4

Ingredients:

- ❖ 1-pint cherry tomatoes
- ❖ 1 package fresh mozzarella balls
- ❖ Fresh basil leaves
- ❖ Balsamic glaze for drizzling

Instructions:

1. Skewer a tomato, mozzarella ball, and basil leaf on toothpicks.
2. Drizzle with balsamic glaze.

Nutritional Information:

120 calories, 5g carbs, 8g protein, 8g fat, 2g fiber.

Experience the classic Italian flavors in a heart-healthy way with these delicious Caprese skewers.

Air-Popped Popcorn with Herbs

Cooking Time: 5 minutes

Serving: 3

Ingredients:

- ❖ 1/2 cup popcorn kernels
- ❖ 1 tablespoon olive oil
- ❖ Dried herbs (rosemary, thyme) for seasoning

Instructions:

1. Pop the corn kernels using an air popper.
2. Drizzle with olive oil, sprinkle with herbs, and toss.

Nutritional Information:

80 calories, 15g carbs, 2g protein, 2g fat, 3g fiber.

Enjoy a guilt-free movie night with air-popped popcorn seasoned with aromatic herbs.

Avocado and Black Bean Salad

Preparation Time: 15 minutes

Serving: 2

Ingredients:

- ❖ 1 avocado (diced)
- ❖ 1 cup black beans (canned, drained)
- ❖ 1/2 cup corn kernels (fresh or frozen)
- ❖ Fresh lime juice for dressing

Instructions:

1. Mix avocado, black beans, and corn in a bowl.
2. Drizzle with lime juice and toss.

Nutritional Information:

230 calories, 30g carbs, 9g protein, 10g fat, 10g fiber.

Elevate your snack time with this avocado and black bean salad, a nutrient-rich and satisfying treat.

Rice Cake with Cottage Cheese and Berries

Preparation Time: 5 minutes

Serving: 1

Ingredients:

- ❖ 1 rice cake (whole grain)
- ❖ 1/2 cup low-fat cottage cheese
- ❖ Mixed berries for topping

Instructions:

1. Spread cottage cheese on the rice cake.
2. Top with mixed berries.

Nutritional Information:

120 calories, 20g carbs, 8g protein, 2g fat, 3g fiber.

Transform a simple rice cake into a delicious and balanced snack with cottage cheese and fresh berries.

Zucchini Chips

Cooking Time: 30 minutes

Serving: 2

Ingredients:

- ❖ 2 medium zucchinis (sliced)
- ❖ 1 tablespoon olive oil
- ❖ Garlic powder and paprika for seasoning

Instructions:

1. Toss zucchini slices with olive oil, garlic powder, and paprika.
2. Bake until crispy.

Nutritional Information:

90 calories, 10g carbs, 2g protein, 6g fat, 3g fiber.

Swap out potato chips for these crispy and flavorful zucchini chips, a heart-healthy alternative.

Bruschetta with Whole Grain Toast

Preparation Time: 15 minutes

Serving: 4

Ingredients:

- ❖ 4 slices whole grain bread
- ❖ 2 cups cherry tomatoes (diced)
- ❖ 1/4 cup fresh basil (chopped)
- ❖ 1 clove garlic (minced)

Instructions:

1. Toast bread slices.
2. Mix tomatoes, basil, and garlic, spoon over the toasted bread.

Nutritional Information:

120 calories, 20g carbs, 5g protein, 2g fat, 4g fiber.

Indulge in the simplicity of bruschetta on whole grain toast, a classic and heart-healthy appetizer or snack.

CHAPTER 5

SOUPS AND STEWS

Tomato Basil Quinoa Soup

Cooking Time: 30 minutes

Serving: 4

Ingredients:

- ❖ 1 can low sodium diced tomatoes.
- ❖ 1/2 cup quinoa (rinsed)
- ❖ 1 onion (chopped)
- ❖ 3 cups low-sodium vegetable broth

Instructions:

1. Combine tomatoes, quinoa, onion, and vegetable broth in a pot.
2. Simmer until quinoa is cooked, garnish with fresh basil.

Nutritional Information:

180 calories, 30g carbs, 7g protein, 2g fat, 5g fiber.

Enjoy the robust flavors of tomato and basil in this nourishing quinoa soup, a wholesome and hearty-friendly option.

Minestrone with Whole Wheat Pasta

Cooking Time: 45 minutes

Serving: 8

Ingredients:

- ❖ 1 cup whole wheat pasta
- ❖ 1 can low-sodium kidney beans (drained)
- ❖ 1 zucchini (diced)
- ❖ 1 cup green beans (cut)
- ❖ 4 cups low-sodium vegetable broth

Instructions:

1. Cook pasta separately.
2. Combine cooked pasta, beans, zucchini, green beans, and vegetable broth in a pot. Simmer until vegetables are tender.

Nutritional Information:

250 calories, 45g carbs, 10g protein, 2g fat, 8g fiber.

Delight in a classic minestrone soup with the added goodness of whole wheat pasta, creating a heart-healthy and satisfying meal.

Butternut Squash and Apple Bisque

Cooking Time: 35 minutes

Serving: 6

Ingredients:

- ❖ 1 medium butternut squash (peeled and cubed)
- ❖ 2 apples (peeled and chopped)
- ❖ 1 onion (chopped)
- ❖ 4 cups low-sodium vegetable broth

Instructions:

1. Sauté onions; add squash, apples, and broth.
2. Simmer until squash is tender. Blend until smooth.

Nutritional Information:

180 calories, 40g carbs, 3g protein, 1g fat, 8g fiber.

Indulge in the velvety richness of butternut squash and apple bisque, a comforting and heartwarming soup.

Spinach and White Bean Stew

Cooking Time: 30 minutes

Serving: 4

Ingredients:

- ❖ 2 cans low-sodium white beans (drained)
- ❖ 1 onion (chopped)
- ❖ 3 cups fresh spinach
- ❖ 2 cloves garlic (minced)

Instructions:

1. Sauté onions and garlic; add white beans and spinach.
2. Simmer until spinach is wilted.

Nutritional Information:

210 calories, 35g carbs, 15g protein, 1g fat, 8g fiber.

Elevate your stew game with this spinach and white bean combination, a nutrient-packed and low-sodium option.

Barley and Mushroom Soup

Cooking Time: 40 minutes

Serving: 6

Ingredients:

- ❖ 1 cup pearl barley
- ❖ 1-pound mushrooms (sliced)
- ❖ 1 onion (diced)
- ❖ 4 cups low-sodium vegetable broth

Instructions:

1. Cook barley separately.
2. Sauté onions and mushrooms; add cooked barley and vegetable broth. Simmer until flavors meld.

Nutritional Information:

220 calories, 40g carbs, 10g protein, 2g fat, 8g fiber.

Experience the heartiness of barley and mushrooms in this wholesome and satisfying soup.

Cabbage and Chickpea Soup

Cooking Time: 35 minutes

Serving: 4

Ingredients:

- ❖ 1/2 head green cabbage (shredded)
- ❖ 1 can low-sodium chickpeas (drained)
- ❖ 1 carrot (sliced)
- ❖ 4 cups low-sodium vegetable broth

Instructions:

1. Combine cabbage, chickpeas, carrot, and vegetable broth in a pot.
2. Simmer until vegetables are tender.

Nutritional Information:

170 calories, 30g carbs, 8g protein, 1g fat, 10g fiber.

Savor the simplicity of cabbage and chickpea soup, a low-sodium option rich in fiber and essential nutrients.

Turmeric-infused Carrot Soup

Cooking Time: 25 minutes

Serving: 4

Ingredients:

- ❖ 1-pound carrots (sliced)
- ❖ 1 onion (chopped)
- ❖ 1 teaspoon turmeric
- ❖ 4 cups low-sodium vegetable broth

Instructions:

1. Sauté onions and carrots; add turmeric and vegetable broth.
2. Simmer until carrots are tender. Blend until smooth.

Nutritional Information:

120 calories, 25g carbs, 2g protein, 1g fat, 5g fiber.

Boost your immune system with the anti-inflammatory properties of turmeric in this vibrant carrot soup.

Red Lentil Curry Stew

Cooking Time: 30 minutes

Serving: 6

Ingredients:

- ❖ 1 cup dry red lentils
- ❖ 1 can low-sodium coconut milk
- ❖ 1 onion (chopped)
- ❖ 2 tablespoons curry powder

Instructions:

1. Cook lentils and onions in coconut milk; add curry powder.
2. Simmer until lentils are soft.

Nutritional Information:

240 calories, 35g carbs, 10g protein, 6g fat, 8g fiber.

Indulge in the rich flavors of red lentil curry stew, a protein-packed and heart-healthy option.

Miso Soup with Tofu and Wakame

Cooking Time: 15 minutes

Serving: 4

Ingredients:

- ❖ 4 cups low-sodium vegetable broth
- ❖ 1/2 cup miso paste
- ❖ 1/2 cup tofu (cubed)
- ❖ 1/4 cup dried wakame seaweed

Instructions:

1. Dissolve miso paste in vegetable broth.
2. Add tofu and wakame; simmer until heated through.

Nutritional Information:

120 calories, 15g carbs, 8g protein, 4g fat, 2g fiber.

Embrace the simplicity and umami flavor of miso soup with tofu and wakame, a light and nourishing option.

Cauliflower and Leek Velouté

Cooking Time: 25 minutes

Serving: 4

Ingredients:

- ❖ 1 medium cauliflower (chopped)
- ❖ 2 leeks (sliced)
- ❖ 2 cloves garlic (minced)
- ❖ 4 cups low-sodium vegetable broth

Instructions:

1. Sauté leeks and garlic until softened; add cauliflower and vegetable broth.
2. Simmer until cauliflower is tender. Blend until velvety.

Nutritional Information:

140 calories, 30g carbs, 5g protein, 1g fat, 7g fiber.

Delight in the silky smoothness of cauliflower and leek velouté, a low-sodium soup that combines simplicity with sophistication.

CHAPTER 6

DESSERTS

Chia Seed Pudding with Berries

Preparation Time: 5 minutes (plus chilling time)

Serving: 2

Ingredients:

- ❖ 1/4 cup chia seeds
- ❖ 1 cup unsweetened almond milk
- ❖ 1 tablespoon honey
- ❖ Mixed berries for topping

Instructions:

1. Mix chia seeds, almond milk, and honey; refrigerate overnight.
2. Top with fresh berries before serving.

Nutritional Information:

150 calories, 15g carbs, 5g protein, 8g fat, 7g fiber.

Indulge guilt-free in this nutrient-packed chia seed pudding, a deliciously sweet treat with heart-healthy benefits.

Baked Apple with Cinnamon

Cooking Time: 30 minutes

Serving: 2

Ingredients:

- ❖ 2 apples (cored and sliced)
- ❖ 1 teaspoon cinnamon
- ❖ 1 tablespoon honey

Instructions:

1. Preheat oven; toss apples with cinnamon and honey.
2. Bake until apples are tender.

Nutritional Information:

120 calories, 30g carbs, 1g protein, 0g fat, 5g fiber.

Enjoy the warmth of baked apples sprinkled with cinnamon, a heart-healthy dessert that's both simple and satisfying.

Avocado Chocolate Mousse

Preparation Time: 10 minutes

Serving: 4

Ingredients:

- ❖ 2 ripe avocados
- ❖ 1/4 cup cocoa powder
- ❖ 1/4 cup maple syrup
- ❖ 1 teaspoon vanilla extract

Instructions:

1. Blend avocados, cocoa powder, maple syrup, and vanilla until smooth.
2. Chill before serving.

Nutritional Information:

180 calories, 20g carbs, 3g protein, 12g fat, 8g fiber.

Satisfy your chocolate cravings with this creamy avocado chocolate mousse, a decadent dessert without the guilt.

Frozen Banana Bites

Preparation Time: 15 minutes (plus freezing time)

Serving: 4

Ingredients:

- ❖ 2 bananas (sliced)
- ❖ 1/4 cup almond butter
- ❖ Dark chocolate for dipping (optional)

Instructions:

1. Spread almond butter on banana slices; freeze.
2. Optional: Dip frozen banana bites in melted dark chocolate.

Nutritional Information:

120 calories, 20g carbs, 3g protein, 5g fat, 3g fiber.

Beat the heat with these frozen banana bites, a delightful and potassium-rich dessert for heart health.

Strawberry Yogurt Parfait

Preparation Time: 10 minutes

Serving: 2

Ingredients:

- ❖ 1 cup low-fat Greek yogurt
- ❖ 1 cup fresh strawberries (sliced)
- ❖ 1/4 cup granola (low sugar)

Instructions:

1. Layer yogurt, strawberries, and granola in a glass.
2. Repeat and enjoy.

Nutritional Information:

180 calories, 25g carbs, 15g protein, 2g fat, 4g fiber.

Delight your taste buds with the freshness of strawberries in this heart-healthy yogurt parfait.

Oatmeal Raisin Cookies

Cooking Time: 15 minutes

Serving: 12

Ingredients:

- ❖ 1 cup oats
- ❖ 1/2 cup whole wheat flour
- ❖ 1/2 cup raisins
- ❖ 1/4 cup unsweetened applesauce

Instructions:

1. Mix oats, flour, raisins, and applesauce.
2. Form into cookies; bake until golden.

Nutritional Information:

90 calories, 20g carbs, 2g protein, 1g fat, 3g fiber.

Indulge in the wholesome goodness of oatmeal raisin cookies, a low sodium treats perfect for a sweet tooth.

Peach and Berry Sorbet

Preparation Time: 10 minutes (plus freezing time)

Serving: 4

Ingredients:

- ❖ 2 cups frozen peaches
- ❖ 1 cup mixed berries
- ❖ 1 tablespoon honey

Instructions:

1. Blend frozen peaches, berries, and honey until smooth.
2. Freeze until firm.

Nutritional Information:

100 calories, 25g carbs, 2g protein, 0g fat, 4g fiber.

Cool down with this refreshing peach and berry sorbet, a naturally sweet and low-sodium dessert.

Mango and Coconut Chia Popsicles

Preparation Time: 10 minutes (plus freezing time)

Serving: 6

Ingredients:

- ❖ 1 cup mango chunks (fresh or frozen)
- ❖ 1 cup coconut milk
- ❖ 2 tablespoons chia seeds

Instructions:

1. Blend mango and coconut milk; stir in chia seeds.
2. Pour into popsicle molds and freeze.

Nutritional Information:

120 calories, 15g carbs, 2g protein, 6g fat, 4g fiber.

Stay cool with these tropical mango and coconut chia popsicles, a delightful and heart-healthy frozen treat.

Blueberry Almond Bites

Preparation Time: 20 minutes (plus chilling time)

Serving: 8

Ingredients:

- ❖ 1 cup blueberries
- ❖ 1/2 cup almonds (chopped)
- ❖ 1/4 cup dates (pitted)
- ❖ 1/4 cup shredded coconut (unsweetened)

Instructions:

1. Blend blueberries, almonds, and dates.
2. Form into bites; roll in shredded coconut. Chill.

Nutritional Information:

80 calories, 15g carbs, 2g protein, 4g fat, 3g fiber.

Experience the burst of antioxidants in these blueberry almond bites, a guilt-free and heart-healthy dessert.

CHAPTER 7

21 DAY MEAL PLAN

Day 1:

- ❖ Breakfast: Berry Blast Smoothie
- ❖ Lunch: Lentil and Vegetable Soup
- ❖ Dinner: Grilled Lemon Herb Chicken with Quinoa
- ❖ Dessert: Chia Seed Pudding with Berries

Day 2:

- ❖ Breakfast: Tomato Basil Quinoa Soup
- ❖ Lunch: Greek Salad with Grilled Chicken
- ❖ Dinner: Minestrone with Whole Wheat Pasta
- ❖ Dessert: Avocado Chocolate Mousse

Day 3:

- ❖ Breakfast: Strawberry Yogurt Parfait
- ❖ Lunch: Spinach and White Bean Stew
- ❖ Dinner: Butternut Squash and Apple Bisque
- ❖ Dessert: Baked Apple with Cinnamon

Day 4:

- ❖ Breakfast: Tropical Paradise Smoothie
- ❖ Lunch: Caprese Salad with Whole Grain Toast
- ❖ Dinner: Red Lentil Curry Stew
- ❖ Dessert: Frozen Banana Bites

Day 5:

- ❖ Breakfast: Blueberry Oat Power Smoothie
- ❖ Lunch: Zucchini Noodles with Pesto and Cherry Tomatoes
- ❖ Dinner: Cabbage and Chickpea Soup
- ❖ Dessert: Strawberry Yogurt Parfait

Day 6:

- ❖ Breakfast: Miso Soup with Tofu and Wakame
- ❖ Lunch: Avocado and Black Bean Salad
- ❖ Dinner: Spinach and White Bean Stew
- ❖ Dessert: Oatmeal Raisin Cookies

Day 7:

- ❖ Breakfast: Minty Watermelon Refresher
- ❖ Lunch: Quinoa Salad with Chickpeas and Veggies
- ❖ Dinner: Barley and Mushroom Soup
- ❖ Dessert: Peach and Berry Sorbet

Day 8:

- ❖ Breakfast: Protein Power Smoothie
- ❖ Lunch: Lentil and Vegetable Soup
- ❖ Dinner: Grilled Lemon Herb Chicken with Quinoa
- ❖ Dessert: Chia Seed Pudding with Berries

Day 9:

- ❖ Breakfast: Banana Almond Bliss Smoothie
- ❖ Lunch: Greek Salad with Grilled Chicken
- ❖ Dinner: Minestrone with Whole Wheat Pasta
- ❖ Dessert: Avocado Chocolate Mousse

Day 10:

- ❖ Breakfast: Citrus Zing Smoothie
- ❖ Lunch: Spinach and White Bean Stew
- ❖ Dinner: Butternut Squash and Apple Bisque
- ❖ Dessert: Baked Apple with Cinnamon

Day 11:

- ❖ Breakfast: Blueberry Oat Power Smoothie
- ❖ Lunch: Caprese Salad with Whole Grain Toast
- ❖ Dinner: Red Lentil Curry Stew
- ❖ Dessert: Frozen Banana Bites

Day 12:

- ❖ Breakfast: Mango and Coconut Chia Popsicles
- ❖ Lunch: Zucchini Noodles with Pesto and Cherry Tomatoes
- ❖ Dinner: Cabbage and Chickpea Soup
- ❖ Dessert: Strawberry Yogurt Parfait

Day 13:

- ❖ Breakfast: Minty Watermelon Refresher
- ❖ Lunch: Avocado and Black Bean Salad
- ❖ Dinner: Spinach and White Bean Stew
- ❖ Dessert: Oatmeal Raisin Cookies

Day 14:

- ❖ Breakfast: Peachy Keen Smoothie
- ❖ Lunch: Quinoa Salad with Chickpeas and Veggies
- ❖ Dinner: Barley and Mushroom Soup
- ❖ Dessert: Peach and Berry Sorbet

Day 15:

- ❖ Breakfast: Berry Blast Smoothie
- ❖ Lunch: Lentil and Vegetable Soup
- ❖ Dinner: Tomato Basil Quinoa Soup
- ❖ Dessert: Avocado Chocolate Mousse

Day 16:

- ❖ Breakfast: Protein Power Smoothie
- ❖ Lunch: Quinoa and Roasted Vegetable Bowl
- ❖ Dinner: Cauliflower and Leek Velouté
- ❖ Dessert: Mango and Coconut Chia Popsicles

Day 17:

- ❖ Breakfast: Minty Watermelon Refresher
- ❖ Lunch: Greek Salad with Grilled Chicken
- ❖ Dinner: Spinach and White Bean Stew
- ❖ Dessert: Strawberry Yogurt Parfait

Day 18:

- ❖ Breakfast: Banana Almond Bliss Smoothie
- ❖ Lunch: Caprese Salad with Whole Grain Toast
- ❖ Dinner: Red Lentil Curry Stew
- ❖ Dessert: Frozen Banana Bites

Day 19:

- ❖ Breakfast: Blueberry Oat Power Smoothie
- ❖ Lunch: Zucchini Noodles with Pesto and Cherry Tomatoes
- ❖ Dinner: Cabbage and Chickpea Soup
- ❖ Dessert: Strawberry Yogurt Parfait

Day 20:

- ❖ Breakfast: Mango and Coconut Chia Popsicles
- ❖ Lunch: Avocado and Black Bean Salad
- ❖ Dinner: Tomato Basil Quinoa Soup
- ❖ Dessert: Oatmeal Raisin Cookies

Day 21:

- ❖ Breakfast: Peachy Keen Smoothie
- ❖ Lunch: Quinoa Salad with Chickpeas and Veggies
- ❖ Dinner: Cauliflower and Leek Velouté
- ❖ Dessert: Peach and Berry Sorbet

CONCLUSION

As we reach the final chapter of our culinary adventure through the pages of " LOW SODIUM COOKBOOK FOR CONGESTIVE HEART FAILURE," I want to extend my heartfelt gratitude for joining me on this transformative journey. Together, we've explored the vibrant landscapes of low sodium living, unlocking the secrets to a healthier heart without compromising on the joy of indulging in delectable flavors.

The stories shared, the recipes savored, and the triumphs celebrated within these pages are not just a testament to the power of mindful eating but also a reflection of the resilience of the human spirit. It is my sincere hope that you, dear reader, have found inspiration within these recipes to embark on your own flavorful journey towards better health.

As you step into your kitchen armed with the knowledge and creativity gained from this cookbook, remember that each meal is an opportunity to nurture your body and soul. Embrace the adventure of crafting delicious, heart-healthy dishes, and savor the joy that comes with knowing you're making choices that resonate with the symphony of your well-being.

Your feedback is a crucial note in the melody of our culinary composition. I invite you to share your thoughts, experiences, and any suggestions you may have. Your insights will not only contribute to the refinement of future editions but also serve as a source of inspiration for those who embark on this journey after you.

Remember, this cookbook is a living document—a reflection of a community committed to the pursuit of a healthier, more flavorful life. Your feedback is the thread that weaves us together, creating a tapestry of shared experiences and collective growth.

Whether you've discovered a new favorite recipe, conquered a culinary challenge, or simply found comfort in the words within these pages, your voice matters. Share your thoughts and let us continue this dialogue beyond the boundaries of these recipes. Together, we can create a chorus of positive change, inspiring others to embrace the nourishing power of a low-sodium lifestyle.

Thank you for entrusting me with a seat at your dining table, and I look forward to hearing about the delicious chapters you add to your own culinary story. May your heart be light, your flavors be bold, and your journey be as delightful as the recipes you've discovered in " LOW SODIUM COOKBOOK FOR CONGESTIVE HEART FAILURE."

BONUS CHAPTER

10 LOW-SODIUM SMOOTHIES

Berry Blast Smoothie

Preparation Time: 5 minutes

Serving: 2

Ingredients:

- ❖ 1 cup mixed berries (strawberries, blueberries, raspberries)
- ❖ 1/2 banana
- ❖ 1/2 cup low-fat Greek yogurt
- ❖ 1 cup almond milk (unsweetened)

Instructions:

1. Blend berries, banana, yogurt, and almond milk until smooth.

Nutritional Information:

150 calories, 25g carbs, 8g protein, 3g fat, 5g fiber.

Kickstart your day with the antioxidant power of mixed berries in this heart-healthy smoothie.

Green Goddess Smoothie

Preparation Time: 7 minutes

Serving: 2

Ingredients:

- ❖ 2 cups spinach (fresh)
- ❖ 1/2 cucumber (peeled)
- ❖ 1/2 avocado
- ❖ 1 cup coconut water (unsweetened)

Instructions:

1. Blend spinach, cucumber, avocado, and coconut water until creamy.

Nutritional Information:

180 calories, 15g carbs, 5g protein, 11g fat, 7g fiber.

Embrace the goodness of greens with this refreshing and nutrient-packed green smoothie.

Tropical Paradise Smoothie

Preparation Time: 6 minutes

Serving: 2

Ingredients:

- ❖ 1 cup pineapple chunks
- ❖ 1/2 mango (peeled)
- ❖ 1/2 cup Greek yogurt (low-fat)
- ❖ 1 cup coconut milk (unsweetened)

Instructions:

1. Blend pineapple, mango, yogurt, and coconut milk until smooth.

Nutritional Information:

160 calories, 30g carbs, 6g protein, 3g fat, 4g fiber.

Transport yourself to a tropical paradise with this heart-healthy and delicious smoothie.

Banana Almond Bliss Smoothie

Preparation Time: 5 minutes

Serving: 2

Ingredients:

- ❖ 2 ripe bananas
- ❖ 1/4 cup almonds (raw)
- ❖ 1 tablespoon almond butter
- ❖ 1 cup almond milk (unsweetened)

Instructions:

1. Blend bananas, almonds, almond butter, and almond milk until creamy.

Nutritional Information:

190 calories, 25g carbs, 5g protein, 9g fat, 5g fiber.

Indulge in the creamy and nutty goodness of this banana almond bliss smoothie for heart-healthy satisfaction.

Citrus Zing Smoothie

Preparation Time: 6 minutes

Serving: 2

Ingredients:

- ❖ 1 orange (peeled)
- ❖ 1/2 grapefruit (peeled)
- ❖ 1/2 cup plain yogurt (low-fat)
- ❖ 1 cup water (cold)

Instructions:

1. Blend orange, grapefruit, yogurt, and water until smooth.

Nutritional Information:

140 calories, 30g carbs, 6g protein, 1g fat, 4g fiber.

Revitalize your senses with the zesty burst of citrus in this heart-healthy and refreshing smoothie.

Protein Power Smoothie

Preparation Time: 8 minutes

Serving: 2

Ingredients:

- ❖ 1 scoop vanilla protein powder
- ❖ 1/2 cup strawberries (fresh or frozen)
- ❖ 1/2 banana
- ❖ 1 cup almond milk (unsweetened)

Instructions:

1. Blend protein powder, strawberries, banana, and almond milk until well combined.

Nutritional Information:

200 calories, 20g carbs, 20g protein, 5g fat, 4g fiber.

Fuel your day with the protein-packed goodness of this delicious and heart-healthy smoothie.

Minty Watermelon Refresher

Preparation Time: 5 minutes

Serving: 2

Ingredients:

- ❖ 2 cups watermelon (seedless)
- ❖ 1/4 cup fresh mint leaves
- ❖ 1/2 lime (juiced)
- ❖ 1 cup coconut water (unsweetened)

Instructions:

1. Blend watermelon, mint, lime juice, and coconut water until smooth.

Nutritional Information:

120 calories, 30g carbs, 2g protein, 1g fat, 3g fiber.

Stay hydrated and refreshed with the delightful combination of watermelon and mint in this heart-healthy smoothie.

Blueberry Oat Power Smoothie

Preparation Time: 7 minutes

Serving: 2

Ingredients:

- ❖ 1 cup blueberries (fresh or frozen)
- ❖ 1/4 cup rolled oats.
- ❖ 1/2 cup Greek yogurt (low-fat)
- ❖ 1 cup almond milk (unsweetened)

Instructions:

1. Blend blueberries, oats, yogurt, and almond milk until smooth.

Nutritional Information:

170 calories, 30g carbs, 8g protein, 3g fat, 5g fiber.

Boost your energy levels with the nutritional power of blueberries and oats in this heart-healthy smoothie.

Peachy Keen Smoothie

Preparation Time: 6 minutes

Serving: 2

Ingredients:

- ❖ 2 peaches (pitted and sliced)
- ❖ 1/2 cup cottage cheese (low-fat)
- ❖ 1/4 teaspoon cinnamon
- ❖ 1 cup water (cold)

Instructions:

1. Blend peaches, cottage cheese, cinnamon, and water until creamy.

Nutritional Information:

160 calories, 25g carbs, 8g protein, 3g fat, 4g fiber.

Enjoy the natural sweetness of peaches in this creamy and heart-healthy smoothie.

Carrot Cake Smoothie

Preparation Time: 8 minutes

Serving: 2

Ingredients:

- ❖ 1 cup carrots (shredded)
- ❖ 1/2 cup pineapple chunks
- ❖ 1/4 cup walnuts
- ❖ 1 cup almond milk (unsweetened)

Instructions:

1. Blend carrots, pineapple, walnuts, and almond milk until smooth.

Nutritional Information:

180 calories, 25g carbs, 5g protein, 8g fat, 5g fiber.

Indulge in the flavors of carrot cake in a heart-healthy way with this satisfying and nutritious smoothie.

MEAL PLANNER JOURNAL
WEEKLY PLANNER

MONDAY	TUESDAY

WEDNESDAY	THURSDAY

FRIDAY	SATUREDAY

SUNDAY	NOTE

WEEKLY PLANNER

MONDAY

TUESDAY

WEDNESDAY

THURSDAY

FRIDAY

SATUREDAY

SUNDAY

NOTE

WEEKLY PLANNER

MONDAY	TUESDAY

WEDNESDAY	THURSDAY

FRIDAY	SATUREDAY

SUNDAY	NOTE

WEEKLY PLANNER

MONDAY	TUESDAY

WEDNESDAY	THURSDAY

FRIDAY	SATUREDAY

SUNDAY	NOTE

WEEKLY PLANNER

MONDAY	TUESDAY

WEDNESDAY	THURSDAY

FRIDAY	SATUREDAY

SUNDAY	NOTE

WEEKLY PLANNER

MONDAY	TUESDAY

WEDNESDAY	THURSDAY

FRIDAY	SATUREDAY

SUNDAY	NOTE

WEEKLY PLANNER

MONDAY	TUESDAY

WEDNESDAY	THURSDAY

FRIDAY	SATUREDAY

SUNDAY	NOTE

WEEKLY PLANNER

MONDAY

TUESDAY

WEDNESDAY

THURSDAY

FRIDAY

SATUREDAY

SUNDAY

NOTE

WEEKLY PLANNER

MONDAY	TUESDAY

WEDNESDAY	THURSDAY

FRIDAY	SATUREDAY

SUNDAY	NOTE

WEEKLY PLANNER

MONDAY

TUESDAY

WEDNESDAY

THURSDAY

FRIDAY

SATUREDAY

SUNDAY

NOTE

www.ingramcontent.com/pod-product-compliance
Lightning Source LLC
Chambersburg PA
CBHW082218290526
45794CB00009B/3586